# MY NATURAL CURLS & COILS

A BEGINNER'S GUIDE TO HEALTH BEAUTIFUL MOISTURIZED CURLS AND COILS

NADINE MORRIS

ISBN: 9798849755724

# PREFACE

This is a straight-to-the-point beginner's guide to healthy, beautiful moisturized curly, kinky coily hair. One of the most asked questions that I've been asked over the years from my customers, clients, family, and friends is, how do I keep my hair moisturized? why is my hair always so dry? What am I doing wrong and how do I fix it?

And after being in the natural hair space for over a decade as a natural hair enthusiast, founder and CEO of a natural and organic hair and skincare brand, a natural hair care consultant, and the founder of Embrace your natural texture workshop, I now have an answer for you!

# TABLE OF CONTENTS

## Preface

# MY NATURAL CURLS AND COILS

# INTRODUCTION

After returning to my natural kinky curls over a decade ago I became fascinated, passionate and obsessed with natural hair care, to the point where I would encourage anyone that would listen about returning to their natural roots. In 2015 I started my natural hair care informational Facebook page called, Adesewa Naturalz and there I gave information on natural hair care, products, DIY, and natural hair care regimens to my naturalistas. Fast forward two years later in 2017 out of necessity I created and formulated my product line by the same name Adesewa Naturalz, and since then I have become a Natural hair care consultant, blogger, and Youtuber who started my workshop called "Embrace your natural texture". And just like that here we are today!

In this book, you will learn how to care for your curls and keep them moisturized. If you've wondered why my curly, kinky coily hair always feels so dry and brittle, and you can't seem to figure out what to do to keep your hair moisturized, manageable and healthy. Don't despair help is here! Continue reading as this book will give you the knowledge and insights on how to care for your curls, and how to keep them healthy, beautiful, and moisturized for days.

# Let's talk hair

Years of miseducation have hampered efforts to grow healthy hair in the natural curly kinky coil hair community. Our pro-hair-grease, anti-water beliefs, pressing comb sessions, to some of us getting our first relaxer at age 7 to tight manipulation styling techniques, have damaged our relationship and hair growth efforts.

Of all the different hair types in the world, curly Kinky coily, hair tends to be the dries. Mainly because the natural oil that is produced by our sebaceous gland called sebum does not easily travel down our spiral curls and corkscrew hair pattern as easily as it does for someone with naturally straight hair. Therefore, leaving the rest of our hair very dry.

Other factors can affect the dryness of our hair, such as; the shampoos we use, the types of products we use to style, and our hair's porosity, Health issues and also our environment, can all affect our hair.

## Ditch the Synthetic Products

One of the first things you should do is to stop using some of the OG conventional products like petroleum hair grease and harsh sulfate-filled shampoo. Most shampoos on the market are formulated to strip the hair completely. These cleaners are excellent for naturally straight and relaxed hair, but not so much for kinky curly-coily hair.

Sulfates are of great concern in the sense that they can have too much of a drying effect on your scalp and hair, resulting in excessive stripping away of naturally occurring proteins and oils.

I've found that a great natural alternative to sulfate shampoo is Organic African black soap.

# The Scalp

Scalp care is important. The scalp is the birthplace of hair so keeping it in proper condition will provide an optimal environment for the follicles to produce quality hair. If your scalp is not cleaned regularly this can be a breeding ground for fungi and bacteria if you allow Product buildup, dirt, and oil to sit there for too long. Whether you wear wigs, weaves, or braids always ensure that your scalp is kept clean at all times.

Ensure that your hair follicles are being nourished with plant-based natural and essential oil mix to help moisturize your scalp. Especially if you suffer from dry scalp issues. Regular scalp massage not only feels great, but it also stimulates the hair follicles and encourages hair growth.

Avoid using petroleum aka hair grease or mineral oil on your scalp, these are some of the synthetic products that does not nourish your scalp, and overtime blocks hydration and moisture from the scalp,

One of the proven facts of natural hair is that curly, kinky coily hair thrives when using natural and organic moisturizing ingredients.

## Keep it Moisturized

Oil is not a moisturizer. A moisturizer must have water or Aloe vera juice listed as one of the first two ingredients in the product list. The first five ingredients on the ingredients list are the most dominant in the product, so be sure that the ingredients are derived from a natural source.

# What's My Hair's Porosity

Hair Porosity – This is your hair's ability to absorb and hold on to moisture. There are three levels of hair porosity, Low Medium, and high porosity.

Low porosity hair does not easily allow moisture in or out of the hair. Strands have a tightly bound cuticle layer with overlapping scales. Low Porosity hair is more prone to product buildup, especially if you are using synthetic products that don't absorb into the hair easily. Low porosity hair can also feel habitually dry at times mainly because of this reason.

Medium Porosity hair allows the right amount of moisture in and out of the hair. This hair porosity needs the least amount of maintenance; it holds styles better and is not normally very dry.

High Porosity hair is usually damaged by chemicals like permanent color treatment, heat damage, or relaxers. When this happens the cuticle has gaps and or holds that make it easy to absorb moisture but just as easily loses moisture. High porosity hair is more prone to frizz, and sealants like thick oils and or heavier butter are needed to help seal the hair to help keep the moisture in the hair longer.

# Characteristics of hair porosity types

Some of the characteristics of Low porosity hair are that it takes longer to dry after wetting, is prone to single strand knots and product build-up, shrinkage is very close to the scalp and it takes a little more effort to stretch.

Medium porosity hair characteristics are that it absorbs and hold on to product well and stays moisturized for at least a couple of days, it gets moderate tangles and knots, and it will stretch with some effort, (shrinkage is not as cumbersome as low porosity hair) and medium porosity hair also holds on to styles fairly well.

High porosity hair tends to dry quickly after being wet, it tangles easily and is prone to breakage whenever tension is applied whether the hair is wet or dry.

# What's My Hair Type

| | Hair Type 2 - Wavy | | Hair Type 3 - Curly | | Hair Type 4 – Kinky Coily |
|---|---|---|---|---|---|
| 2a | Curl shape between straight and curly<br>Fine/Thin hair<br>Easily styled | 3a | "S" curl shape<br>Loose curls<br>Easily straightened | 4a | Tight "S" curls densely packed together<br>Wiry to fine texture<br>More fragile than other hair types |
| 2b | Medium texture hair<br>Little resistance to styling<br>Tendency to Frizz | 3b | Numerous springy curls<br>Requires work to straighten<br>Coarse Texture | 4b | "Z" curl shape, bends in sharp angles<br>Cotton like hair<br>Can be wiry/coarse and fine/thin and is fragile |
| 2c | Coarse hair<br>Resists styling<br>Frizzes | 3c | Tight corkscrew curls<br>Kinky curls densely packed<br>Fine texture<br>Harder to style than 3a or 3b | 4c | Ziggly hair with no definition densely packed<br>Dry and very fragile<br>Thick and coarse or thin and soft |

As I always say good hair is the hair you grow naturally, but great hair is the result of how you care for it.

Without putting in the time and effort, curly, kinky coily hair can become very dry and brittle, and dry and brittle hair leads to breakage and split ends. The truth is all hair types are manageable once you have the patience, find the right products, and develop your routine.

Let's talk more about some of the internal and external factors that can affect hair growth and the quality of your hair. Some of the external factors can be; environmental such as harsh winter weather, Hair care practices such as chemical treatment, products we use, and sometimes just normal wear and tear from pulling or brushing too hard are all factors.

Some internal factors are; genetics example, male or female pattern baldness, health issues such as low Iron, thyroid issues, medication, hormones, diet, and nutrition are all factors that can affect your hair growth and quality of hair.

# Do I need to wash often?

Let's debunk the hair myth, how often should curly, kinky coily, hair be washed? Let me put it this way. Remember your hair is like a plant, it needs water and nourishment to grow. I say wash as needed. Your lifestyle will play a role in this as well. But ideally, 7 to 10 days is good but you can get away with washing it once every 14 days if you don't have any scalp issues or excessive product build-up. I find that for individuals with Locs that maintain a loc routine, 2-4 weeks typically works for them. Washing your hair helps to prevent hair and scalp dryness, clogged scalp pores, and product build-up all of which can later develop into scalp issues if not kept in check.

## TLC for my Strands

Regular deep conditioning is a MUST for kinky curly, coily hair. Deep conditioning helps to prevent breakage, it replaces moisture loss and improves your hair's elasticity. It is especially important for those with dry, damaged, brittle, or color-treated hair. Most importantly, when you deep condition your hair, you help restore luster, shine, strength, and softness into your hair.

Keep in mind that a hair regimen for chemically treated hair must always work to restore the hair's moisture to protein balance by reinforcing the hair's protein structure.

# Let's Go Deep

What type of deep conditioner should I use? The type of deep conditioner you use for your hair will depend on your hair texture and the state of your hair. For example, dry hair will require a conditioner that is formulated for softness and moisture.

***Moisturizing deep conditioners*** with lots of oils and emollient, and moisturizing properties should be used for hair that is very dry and requires softening.

***Re-constructor's deep conditioners*** may contain a lot of protein and can be used on hair that is fine, limp, and on damaged or color-treated hair a little bit more regularly than hair that is not.

***Protein deep conditioners*** are also called treatments, I call the protein deep conditioner my heavy hitters. A protein treatment should contain hydrolyzed proteins, as these protein molecule structures penetrate and attach to your hair in the areas that are weak to help strengthen the hair by hardening the hair's cuticle layer and

putting a protective barrier around the hair. Protein treatments also help to improve your hair's elasticity and make it less prone to breakage.

Protein treatment can be used once per month or every 6-8 weeks depending on the condition and feel of your hair. Some protein treatments (depending on the brand) can cause your hair to feel very hard, and in cases like these, you will need to follow up with a moisturizing deep conditioner.

Be careful not to overuse protein in your hair care regimen, otherwise, your hair will get dry and hard, and this will lead to breakage.

___**Note**___: always focus the conditioner on the length of your hair shaft and the ends of your hair; avoid applying it to your scalp. Always rinse hair with cool water after the conditioning process. Cool water helps to close the hair's cuticle.

***Hot Oil treatments*** are especially great for curly, kinky coily hair. Use plant-based oils that are hair approved for your hot oil treatments. Once you have incorporated hot oil treatment into your regimen and start to do it consistently you will begin to notice, stronger roots, less frizz, healthier scalp, moisture retention, less breakage, shine and luster, decrease in split ends, and fewer single strand knots.

If you live in a colder climate, hot oil treatments are great to do in the winter months.

## Time to Style

After the shampoo and conditioning process follow up with the WLCO method, layering your products will allow your hair to stay moisturized for a longer time. Curly, kinky coily hair needs Moisture! Moisture! Moisture!

Now let's break down WLCO method which is layering your products for longer moisture retention, this method consists of four main steps and products: spritz the hair with water, apply your leave-in-conditioner, next your moisturizing hair cream or styling cream, and then last oil of your choice. Layering your products will also help to guard against friction and other damaging elements rubbing against your hair and causing breakage and this method also helps to prevent excessive dryness.

## Part 1: Pro Tips

Always clarify your hair and scalp before starting a new hair care regimen. Using a great clarifying shampoo or a bentonite clay hair mask will do wonders for your hair. What this does is give you a fresh clean slate for your new products to thoroughly absorb into your hair strands and be effective.

when styling your hair especially Low and Medium porosity hair spritz hair with warm water and scrunch water into the hair before applying your products. Warm water will help to open up your hair's cuticle and help your hair to absorb the products better.

For my Low porosity naturals, be sure to use lightweight and easily absorbable moisturizers and oils, this will help to prevent excess product buildup on your stands.

Always moisturize curly, kinky coily hair

in small to medium manageable sections, (this will be depending on the density of your hair). Moisturizing in sections will allow for every strand of hair to be thoroughly moisturized and coated with products. Also pay special attention to the ends of your hair, because this is the oldest and driest part of your hair.

Never detangle dry hair. Make sure your hair is slightly damp before detangling. To minimize painful detangling use your fingers first, before using a wide tooth comb or detangling brush.

Start detangling from the ends of your hair and work your way up to the root. Proper detangling reduces hair breakage.

Avoid over-brushing your hair, especially when it's dry, as this will only cause frizz.

Avoid excessive heat styling. Heat styling over a period of time will cause heat damage.

# 14 Must-Have Tools for Your Natural Hair Journey

Having these tools in your must-haves for your curly, kinky coily hair is essential to making your wash days and maintaining your styles easier.

## Spray Bottle

Is great for wetting your hair while styling. It's also beneficial when you have to refresh your hair without drenching it. You can also add your DIY moisturizers to it. It's best to work on Damp hair before applying your moisturizer.

## Wide Tooth Comb

A wide tooth comb will help you to detangle without causing excessive breakage. The spaces in this comb will allow you to move through your hair without ripping out your ends.

## Thermal Heat Cap OR Hooded dryer/ Hair steamer

A Thermal heat Cap is another great tool for your curly, kinky coily hair. Adding heat to your deep conditioning sections will help the nourishing ingredients penetrate your strands better. This is a tool you'll use frequently in your natural hair regimen, especially if you deep condition regularly.

## Detangling Brush

You want to ensure you're able to detangle easily and faster on wash days. A good detangling brush should do an amazing job at removing tangles. You want to use this with a product that has a lot of slip! always finger detangle before using this brush just to make sure you won't rip your hair out.

# Rat Tail Comb

Are pretty useful! If you need to part your hair neatly, then this is the perfect tool to use.

You can also use this comb to smooth out the ends of my hair (after detangling) whenever you are doing a twist-out or braid-out style. A rat tail comb is also great for starter locs and comb coils.

# Croc' Clips

If you have longer and thicker hair, you will need something that would hold your hair in place.

These clips make sectioning your hair so much easier and it'll help you to focus on one section at a time without some strands getting in the way. So, if you have a hard time finding clips to hold your hair OR they are always breaking, then this is a great tool for your natural hair.

# Hair Ties

When it comes to wearing a high puff, you will need a great hair tie. Goodie has some great ones. Stay away from the ones that have the metal clamps and the ones that are not smooth as these will cause breakage.

# Satin Bonnet/Pillowcase

Wearing a satin bonnet or sleeping on a satin pillowcase will ensure your natural hair is protected for the next day, hopefully! avoid sleep or tying your hair with cotton, as cotton will absorb moisture.

Satin will keep the moisture in your hair, minimize unwanted frizz, and ensure your curls stay intact. I love wearing bonnets; however, a pillowcase will provide the same benefits!

## Diffuser

Investing in a diffuser is perfect for the colder months when you want to achieve a wash-and-go style. A diffuser can be used to dry your hair faster, cut down on shrinkage, and provide volume for your curls.

## Applicator Bottle

An applicator bottle is a perfect tool for natural hair when it comes to doing hot oil treatments, pre-pooing, or simply adding oil to your scalp.

## Bobby Pins

Bobby pins can be used to hold flyaway hair in place while keeping your style looking cute. There are also some beautiful and creative hair accessories for natural hair.

## Hair Pick

Another tool for natural hair I feel is necessary if you're looking for volume is a hair pick. You can add volume to your styles by focusing the hair pick on your roots. The last thing you want is to lose any definition you achieved and cause frizz. A hair pick will help you achieve the big, voluminous hair you're looking for!

## T-shirt Towel OR Microfiber Towel

Cotton T-shirt are soft and won't catch on the hair strands. Microfiber towel has fast-drying properties, and microfiber towels are also not as rough as other types of towels. They also absorb the wetness without getting too wet themselves.

## Shears

The last tool I recommend for your natural hair journey is a pair of shears. If you want to trim your hair at home or 'dust' your ends once in a while, it's important to invest in good-quality shears.

Using household scissors to cut your hair won't give you the perfect ends you're looking for. Shears are sharper than household scissors and will provide a precise cut.

## Protective style

Protective styles are great especially when you need a break from styling your hair; However, remember that proactive styles are for "protecting your hair", whether it be from environmental elements such as seasonal winter weather or while on vacation. So, the rule of thumb is, do not neglect your hair while wearing a protective style! especially if you will be wearing that style for several weeks. Still keep your hair and scalp healthy and clean so that you can retain all the length from your new growth.

Avoid wearing high-stress hairstyles for long periods. Tight ponytails and tight braids can look chic, but they also put a lot of stress on your hair and scalp. Over time, they can create crimps and breakage in the hair. This can also stress the hair follicles, cause thinning along the hairline, and cause traction alopecia.

**_Note_**: Always allow your hair to rest for a few weeks before you put in another protective style.

## To Trim or Not to Trim

Trim your split ends as needed, some naturals opt for 2-3 times per year, others don't want to ever see a set of shears ever again. Even healthy hair is prone to getting spit ends and single strand knots, so be sure to check your hair for them regularly; the longer you leave your split ends unchecked, the further damage it causes. The number of times per year to get a trim is not written in stone, the best thing to do in this case is to listen to your hair.

Nevertheless, having your ends trimmed will allow your hair to grow healthier and thus longer.

Don't rely on "split end mending" serum, because they are only temporary fixes; they are not permanent and will not mend or fix your split ends. The only thing that works is trimming them.

# Part 2: Pro Tips

## How do you know when my hair needs a trim?

You will have a lot of single strand knots, your ends will tangle easily, and they never look, stay or feel moisturized. it won't curl or hold definition as the rest of your hair. Your ends will look thin and stringy whenever you do your twist, and your hair will lack volume, as a result of you holding on to dead ends.

## How do you know when my hair needs moisture?

If your wet hair feels rough, hard, and tangly, or if your hair does not stretch much before braking, you need to do more moisturizing deep conditioning.

### *How do I know when my hair needs a protein treatment?*

If your wet hair feels weak, gummy, and limp or your hair has no elasticity meaning it stretches too far before breaking, do a protein treatment.

## Let's Seal it and tie it with a Bow

Last but not least, there is no quick fix or magic pill that will give you healthy, beautiful, moisturized hair. You have to put in the work! Being consistent, along with healthy hair care practices, quality products, and a healthy lifestyle are all keys to retaining your length and having healthy thriving hair…

Because as I always say "good hair is the hair you grow naturally, but great hair is a result of how you care for it".

## About the Author

Nadine Morris is a natural hair care consultant, blogger and the founder and CEO of Adesewa Naturalz, a natural and organic hair and skin care product line in Canada. After returning to her natural roots over a decade ago and falling in love with her natural curls and coils, this love led her to create a space for herself and a business serving the natural hair community. Since 2015 she has been doing what she loves best, formulating beauty products and sharing her knowledge with clients, customers, family and friends.

# MY NATURAL CURLS AND COILS